MIKE'S
HOW TO GUIDE FOR
SUSTAINABLE WEIGHT LOSS!

MICHAEL BAKER

Copyright © 2022 Michael Baker

All rights reserved. No part of this publication may be reproduced, distributed, or transmitted in any form or by any means, including photocopying, recording, or other electronic or mechanical methods, without the prior written permission of the publisher, except in the case of brief quotations embodied in critical reviews and certain other noncommercial uses permitted by copyright law. For permission requests, contact mikessustainableweightloss@gmail.com.

I must start out by saying this first. I am not a board-certified dietician nor am I a health expert. If you have food allergies, please review my suggestions, and make sure there aren't any allergy issues for you personally. You should always review your plan with your doctor.

I'm a normal guy, who had some serious cardiac health issues occur a year ago at the young age of 35, "most likely due to the covid vaccine," as it is written in my medical record.

I believe the seriousness was also partially due to not taking care of myself or my diet over the years.

I have a wife and three young children I'd like to watch grow up. I realized after my near-death experience, and feeling terrible for many months afterwards, it was time to make changes and take better care of myself for me and for them.

Over the last many years my wife and I have tried various fad diets, crash diets, no carb diets, juice diets, cleanse diets, keto, and expensive diet systems/programs just to name a few.

But, like so many others in the world, none of these methods were sustainable long-term solutions. The ideas and changes I have made are not rocket science or novel ideas either. But it takes a strong WHY. It takes dedication, drive, and a lot of effort on YOUR part to stay on track.

As a result of my health issues, I implemented changes to my food intake and have seen rather dramatic results over the last 10+ Months. I have lost 65lbs, am down from a 42 waist to a 32, plus, my shirts are XL vs XXL! I continue to see improvements every single week.

I rarely feel starving, as I eat frequently and plentiful. I have more energy and I now seriously enjoy eating healthily, after sticking with the lifestyle changes as described below.

Not to mention, everything is easier without the watermelon in my abdomen. I also have way more energy and I am no longer making excuses to eat and drink mindlessly.

It is your small choices daily that snowball over time. Like all things in life, if you consistently make good choices, over time you will see good results. If you consistently make bad choices, over time, you will see bad results.

My goal is to motivate you to make the changes you need to make. I want to help you achieve your weight loss goals, feel more energetic and be healthier overall.

My results may not be typical, and you may not see the same results, but rest assured if you are making good choices daily, you will see some sort of positive return to your life and how you feel overall.

This is not another Fad Diet, Crash Diet, Starving yourself Diet or another expensive Diet Program. I am simply giving you the tools to lose weight and achieve your weight loss goals and it is up to you to make it happen.

- **You** must eat intentionally and thoughtfully, for the purpose of giving your body the right fuel for your desired outcome.

- No more eating your next snack because you're stressed, or upset, or overtired or because it just tastes so damn good.

- Follow the steps ahead to consistently lose weight and lose it healthily. You can maintain your weight loss once you've hit your target weight by sticking with your new habits.

- You will seriously enjoy all the great nutritious foods you are going to be eating and your portion sizes will be correct moving forward to help you keep the weight off.

- Like anything else in life, **you** have to implement, and **you** have to want to change things for **yourself** first.
- Only **you** can decide what to put in your mouth.
- Your **why** has to be powerful to drive your will power to change.

The statements ahead have not been evaluated by any dietary professionals and are based on my opinion and own personal experiences. I have not been paid by anyone to put my list of recommendations out for you to digest. Yes, pun intended.

MY 10 STEPS

1. Determine your Basic Metabolic Rate (BMR) by utilizing an Online Calculator. Like the one that can be found by searching BMR Calculator on google. Find one that takes into consideration your activity level, age, height, and weight and adjust your total daily calories accordingly.
2. For the First three months at least, you will need to count calories of everything you consume.

3. Count your total calories and keep it slightly above your recommended BMR.
4. Your drinks also count toward your Daily Caloric Intake, Except for Water.
5. Drink as much water as you can throughout the day. It will keep you full and hydrated.
6. You must read nutritional facts on everything and be sure to adhere to the portion sizes, plus, understand what the ingredients are. You want High Protein, High Dietary Fiber, Low Saturated Fats and Low Carbohydrates.
7. Avoid drinks that have a lot of Carbs (including alcohol for a while) but also avoid the drinks that claim "No sugar" because they add in fake

sugar substitutes like Sucralose & Aspartame.

8. **Plan** your daily food and leave your house prepared for the whole day with healthy snacks like fresh fruit, fresh veggies, cheese sticks, premade salad and protein bars with low net carbs and high fiber.

9. Plan to eat every 3 Hours and keep each snack healthy and between 100 and 250 Calories so you won't feel hangry or sluggish throughout the day.

10. Full Meals should not be any more than 750 calories at a time and be made up of, Protein & Vegetables. Eat low carb, or complex carbs like brown rice or sweet potatoes when you eat Carbs.

MORE TIPS TO STAY ON TRACK:

- Focus your food planning on eating Protein and Veggies with complex carbs. Protein and Veggies, and yes you guessed it, Protein and Veggies.
- Take a Daily Multivitamin pill in the morning.
- Proteins like fresh Chicken breast, ground turkey, fish, pea protein powders to mix with water or almond milk are the proteins I am referring to. Red meat once in a while is OK, but not every day.
- Veggies – **All fresh, unbattered and unbuttered**
- **NO Fast Food or Soda!!!** Unless they serve Salads with un-fried protein and low carb balsamic dressing. If you go out to

eat, find a meal less than 800 calories or have a salad. Also, when you eat salad, don't slobber the healthy salad with a creamy high calorie/high fat dressing and have 25 croutons on it. That defeats the purpose of having a salad.

- Have Low net carb wraps on hand to put your veggies and proteins in for a quick satisfying snack or meal. NO MAYO. Guacamole or Balsamic Vinaigrette dressing or low carb option only.
- Move around more doing any additional activity you can. It will get easier as you shed pounds and your body will feel better and more energetic as you improve your overall health

- **Think of food as fuel for your body. You're not eating your fuel for enjoyment. After doing this for a few months you will change your relationship with food, and you will enjoy eating salads and all the other healthy options that are out there.**
- We all stress eat when we aren't focused on what we are trying to accomplish. You can stop doing this, if you prepare and have the right choices available, when you have the urge.
- If you eat Pizza, because you know we all like pizza, have a half plate of salad and only one piece of pizza. If you get a

burger, try and eat half the bun or no bun!

- Use an Air Fryer or Cook on the grill with dry rub spices. Lemon Pepper Chicken is one of my favorite dry rubs.

MY SUGGESTED SNACKS TO HAVE AVAILABLE:

- American or Provolone Cheese
- Bell Peppers, any color
- Broccoli
- Carrots
- Celery Sticks
- Cheese Sticks
- Cucumbers
- Dry Spices— load up your entrees and snacks with garlic, pepper, basil, oregano, or

everything bagel seasoning, it makes everything delicious.
- Eggs, hard boiled, over easy or scrambled
- Fresh fruit- any berries, any apples, any citrus or any melons - Eat fresh fruit frequently
- Grilled Chicken breast or air fryer chicken breast to use on salads or in wraps
- Guacamole (tubs or squeeze container style)
- Hummus
- Low Carb wrap options
- Medium Salsa and Guacamole are great additions to just about anything, Don't use Ketchup or other condiments.
- One Serving of Nutella on its own or with the Peanut Butter (if no allergies)

- One serving of Peanut Butter on its own (if no allergies)
- One slice of whole wheat bread with a serving of Peanut Butter on it (if no allergies)
- Pepperoncini
- Pickles
- Pirate Booty Air puffs
- Plain Yogurt or Cottage Cheese
- Premade Fresh Salads from your local supermarket with balsamic dressing or low carb option.
- Protein Bars with Low Net Carbs – I recommend Quest Protein Bars
- Protein Powder- Orgain, Muscle Milk, or Arbonne options are good
- Romaine Lettuce OR Iceberg Lettuce

- Shredded Mozzarella or Mexican Blend Cheese
- Skinny Pop 100 Calorie bags
- Sliced Baked Honey Ham
- Sliced Turkey Breast
- Taboule
- Veggie Straws or Veggie Chips
- Whole wheat bread toast, with Avocado and everything seasoning on it

MY DAILY MENU EXAMPLE:

BREAKFAST:

- Coffee with Almond Milk Or Low Carb Energy Drink (my preference is Reign or Redbull)
- Water
- 1 or 2 Quest Protein Bars OR Three Eggs with Salsa and Guacamole

LUNCH:

- Water
- 1 Premade Salad with protein on it and Balsamic dressing
- 1 Quest Protein Bar

Dinner:

- Water
- Freshly cooked dry rubbed Chicken Breast cooked in an Air Fryer or on the Grill
- 1 small serving of Brown Rice based on serving size on box
- Your choice of a fresh vegetable (I used Frozen microwaveable veggies too, not canned)
- Have a fresh salad with balsamic dressing as an extra side

Snacks:

- Water
- 1-2 String Cheese Stick
- 2 Eggs with Guacamole and Salsa as toppings

- 2 Apples
- A Handful of Raspberries and Blueberries
- Half a sliced cucumber with Italian or Balsamic dressing
- Low Carb Wrap with Romaine lettuce, 1 piece of American cheese and 2 slices of Turkey or Ham
- 1 Slice Whole Wheat Bread with Avocado Spread and Everything Seasoning
- Protein Shake with Almond Milk or Water

Try to drink half of your body weight in ounces of water every day. This will keep you full and hydrated.

If you get bored of any of the food options, get creative and change them out for another healthy choice to keep it interesting. Incorporate Fruit, Veggies and Protein into your new option.

IF you are going to exceed your daily calories, make sure you are exceeding it with Fresh Fruit,

Fresh Veggies or Protein – not chips, cookies, pie, or cake.

ADDITIONAL NOTES:

If you don't have it in you to plan out your meals, use a reputable local meal prep service to get your healthy premade meals from. They should be balanced between protein, veggies, and carbs. They should be made fresh and be freezable, to take out and microwave as needed to supplement your other healthy food choices.

If you're struggling with low energy, I highly recommend making sure your hormones are all in check by visiting health care providers that deal with hormones and other health aspects. Some Internal Medicine doctors may not even think to look at these areas of your health.

You can still eat a Pasta, Pizza, and yes, you can still eat Ice cream. The Key is don't OVERDO it and DO NOT do it every day. It is OK to treat yourself as you won't sustain your lifestyle changes if you don't enjoy something extra tasty occasionally--- **but don't OVERDO it and DO NOT do it every day.**

This is a journey. As Darren Hardy says, it is your small choices overtime that will Compound (positively or negatively) to make a difference in your life (and on the Scale!)

As you lose weight, you BMR is going to change, so you will need to revisit Step 1 and re-configure your daily intake based on your updated numbers.

Again, I am not a dietary professional but have implemented these changes and have seen dramatic results. I don't promise you will see the same results but I can promise you will see a positive return on your life in one way or another if you make positive choices.

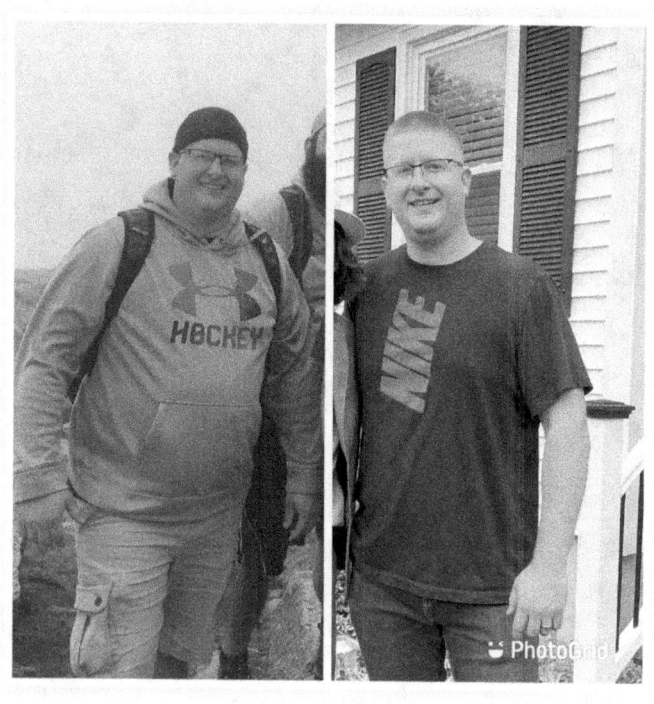

Please share your successes so you too can influence others to join in on your journey with me at:

mikessustainableweightloss@gmail.com

www.ingramcontent.com/pod-product-compliance
Lightning Source LLC
Chambersburg PA
CBHW070322220526
45465CB00013B/2173